YOUR KNOWLEDGE HAS VALUE

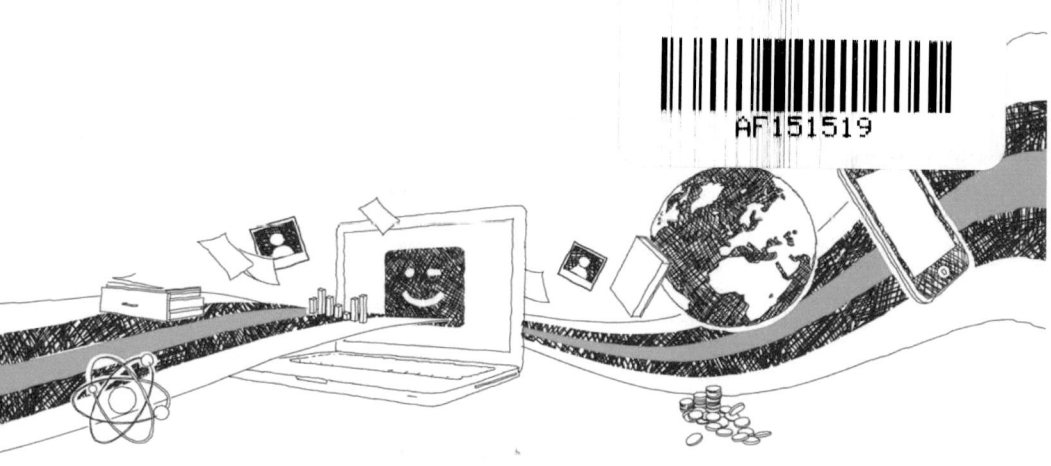
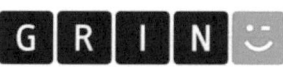

Imprint:

Copyright © 2014 GRIN Verlag, Open Publishing GmbH
Print and binding: Books on Demand GmbH, Norderstedt Germany
ISBN: 978-3-668-02413-7

This book at GRIN:

http://www.grin.com/en/e-book/303791/cardiac-arrest-the-side-effects-of-saving-lifes

Antje Dangel

Cardiac Arrest. The Side Effects of Saving Lifes

A Case Study

GRIN Publishing

GRIN - Your knowledge has value

Since its foundation in 1998, GRIN has specialized in publishing academic texts by students, college teachers and other academics as e-book and printed book. The website www.grin.com is an ideal platform for presenting term papers, final papers, scientific essays, dissertations and specialist books.

Visit us on the internet:

http://www.grin.com/

http://www.facebook.com/grincom

http://www.twitter.com/grin_com

Cardiac Arrest – The Side Effects of Saving Lives

Antje Dangel

University of South Florida

Table of Contents

Introduction

Currently, heart disease remains the leading cause of death while cardiac arrest is one of the most devastating conditions patients and their families have to face. Despite all efforts to explain management of cardiac arrest and implementation of advanced cardiovascular life support (ACLS), survival rates post cardiac arrest remains at 23.9 % in adults and 40.2% in children (AHA, 2012). Nurses undergo extensive ACLS training every two years. While algorithms, administration of emergency drugs, and procedures seem to be followed appropriately, rationales of the latter are often not well understood. In this paper pharmacokinetics and pharmacodynamics, adverse effects of ACLS drugs, drug-drug interactions of intervention drugs, and anticipated long-term adverse effects post cardiac arrest will be discussed. In the case study of JG, the patient went into cardiac arrest on the way to the hospital and he was pronounced after a full code had been performed for three hours. The cause of his cardiac arrest in regards to heart rhythm is unclear and no medical history is available.

ACLS Guidelines

ACLS guidelines, developed by the American Heart Association (AHA) recommend cardiopulmonary resuscitation (CPR) and defibrillation for cardiac arrest secondary to ventricular fibrillation (VF) or ventricular tachycardia (VT). Additionally, pharmacological treatment consists of administering intravenous (IV) vasopressors and anti-arrhythmic drugs (AHA, 2010). Pharmacological management of asystole includes epinephrine administration every 3-5 minutes; the first or second dose of epinephrine may be substituted with vasopressin.

3

Clinical Pharmacology of Emergency Drugs

Emergency drugs have no contraindications as they are intended to prevent premature death; however, as most drugs, emergency drugs react systemically and adverse reactions and possible long-term consequences need to be considered. The following section addresses the pharmacodynamics and pharmacokinetics as well as adverse reactions and disease interactions of epinephrine, vasopressin, amiodarone, and lidocaine.

Vasopressin versus Epinephrine - Amiodarone versus Lidocaine

Pharmacodynamics

Epinephrine, a sympathomimetic catecholamine acting on both alpha and beta-adrenergic receptors, benefits patients during cardiac arrest due to its receptor stimulating properties (FDA, n.d.). Epinephrine's alpha-adrenergic effects lead to systemic vasoconstriction, and subsequently to increased myocardial and cerebral blood flow (AHA, 2000). Epinephrine has a rapid onset and short duration of action with a half-life of 2 minutes (Food and Drug Administration [FDA], n.d.).

Vasopressin, a noradrenergic polypeptide antidiuretic hormone that causes contraction of vascular and other smooth muscles, benefits patients in cardiac arrest due to stimulation of V1 and V2 receptors. Stimulation of V1 receptors leads to peripheral, coronary, and renal vasoconstriction, while stimulation of V2 receptors leads to vasodilation, and subsequent reduction of end-organ hypoperfusion. Vasopressin also leads to increased cerebral blood flow by vasodilation. It is suspected that vasopressin administration during cardiac arrest leads to decreased incidences of long-term neurological damage (Wenzel, 2004). Vasopressin increases systemic vascular resistance and mean arterial pressure, therefore decreases heart rate and cardiac workload (FDA, n.d.). Onset and peak are rapid and half-life is 10-20 minutes.

Amiodarone, a class III antiarrhythmic, benefits patients in cardiac arrest by blocking calcium, sodium and potassium channels, which slows conduction and prolongs refractoriness of the atrioventricular (AV) node. Amiodarone has vasodilatory effects triggering sympathetic activity, which lead to decreased cardiac workload and subsequent decreased myocardial oxygen consumption. Amiodarone has, in comparison with lidocaine, very little negative inotropic activity. IV amiodarone has a rapid onset, half-life in blood plasma is relatively short, exact time is unknown (Giardina & Passman, 2014).

Lidocaine, a class Ib antiarrhythmic drug, benefits patients in cardiac arrest by decreasing depolarization and automaticity of ventricular cells and by increasing ventricular fibrillation threshold. Onset of IV lidocaine is immediate and half-life is 10 minutes (Karch, 2012).

Adverse Reactions

According to the FDA, all ACLS drugs have adverse effects that affect almost all body systems. Most problematic adverse effects include those that affect the cardiovascular and renal system. This is especially true with amiodarone; however, no long-term studies analyzing side effects of short term administration of IV amiodarone exist.

Disease Interaction According to the FDA

Epinephrine should be used with caution and may precipitate underlying heart conditions in patients who have heart disease to include arrhythmias, coronary artery or organic heart disease, or cerebrovascular disease. The use of vasopressin in patients with impaired cardiac response may worsen cardiac output. The use of amiodarone is cautioned when patients present with preexisting conditions including cardiac conduction deficits, pulmonary disease, liver disease, renal impairment, and thyroid disease. Lastly, lidocaine can cause significant problems if severe liver or renal disease, hypovolemia, shock, or heart blocks exists (FDA, n.d.).

Drug-Drug Interactions

According to the FDA (n.d.), epinephrine should not be given in addition to other sympathomimetic drugs in order to avoid additive effects. Cardiac glycosides, digitalis, diuretics, quinidine, and other antiarrhythmics may exacerbate cardiac arrhythmias. Some drugs, including antidepressants, levothyroxine, and antihistamines, may potentiate the effects of epinephrine.

Drugs interacting with vasopressin include catecholamines, indomethacin, ganglionic blocking agents, furosemide, drugs suspected of causing syndrome of inappropriate antidiuretic hormone secretion (SIADH), and drugs suspected of causing diabetes insipidus. Drug-drug interactions include effects related to mediation by V1 receptors resulting in release of calcium, leading to vasoconstriction and stimulation of V2 receptors causing antidiuresis (FDA, n.d.) It is important to note that indomethacin doubles the time to offset vasopressin's effect, while ganglionic blocking agents increase the pressor effect by 20% in healthy patients (FDA, n.d.). Furosemide increases osmolar clearance and urine flow when co-administered with vasopressin (FDA, n.d.)

Giardina & Passman (2014) note that amiodarone is a potent metabolite inhibitor, potentially leading to significant drug interactions. Potential drug class interactions with Amiodarone include beta-blockers (BBs) and calcium channel blockers (CCBs). BBs as well as CCBs cause hypotension, which could be exacerbated by the use of amiodarone. Moreover, amiodarone is over 96% bound to protein; therefore it competes with other highly protein bound drugs to include digoxin and warfarin. Digoxin and INR levels may rise, and frequent lab draws are warranted after initiation of amiodarone therapy.

The FDA notes that lidocaine should be used with caution when co-administered with beta-blockers, H2-antagonists, and other antiarrhythmics due to additive, antagonizing, or toxic effects of drug combination.

Review of Literature

While some studies showed no significant difference in survival to discharge with respect to vasopressin over epinephrine administration during cardiac arrest secondary to VF or PEA, other studies show an increased chance of survival after vasopressin over epinephrine administration if cardiac arrest was brought on by asystole (Wenzel, 2004). Subsequent studies have not confirmed the latter, and Oberweis (2011) suggests that the superiority finding of vasopressin over epinephrine is linked to extreme ischemia and acidosis. A systematic review and meta-analysis conducted by Aung & Htay (2005) concluded that there is no clear advantage of vasopressin over epinephrine in incessant VF as it pertains to return of spontaneous circulation (ROSC.) Stroumpoulis et al. (2008) found that the administration of vasopressin in combination with epinephrine led to drastically improved results in regards to ROSC, but not in regards to survival to discharge rates. Somberg et al. (2002) found that amiodarone was favorable over lidocaine in the treatment of incessant VT, as lidocaine had a 91% drug failure rate compared to a 33% drug failure rate of amiodarone. A recent study conducted by Mauerman et al. (2012) examined amiodarone versus lidocaine and placebo for the prevention of ventricular fibrillation after aortic crossclamping. The study showed that amiodarone decreased the number of shocks needed to cease VF. On the contrary, there was no difference between lidocaine and placebo in

7

the number of required shocks. Body and Brady (2011) performed a thorough review of literature with respect to cardioactive medications in cardiac arrest resuscitation. The authors concluded that insufficient evidence with regards to long-term survival exist; however, study results pertaining to short-term survival were promising and given the risk of death during cardiac arrests, continuation of current algorithms was suggested (Body &Brady, 2011).

Consideration of Other Commonly Prescribed Cardiac Drugs

All drugs used for the management of cardiac arrest interact in some way with commonly prescribed cardiac medication. This is due to the nature of their alpha and beta effects as well as the antidiuretic property of vasopressin and the potent inhibition of drug metabolites by amiodarone. Often times, patients who go into cardiac arrest self-administer an array of medications affecting multiple body systems. Commonly prescribed medications include diuretics, alpha and beta blockers, calcium channel blockers, anticoagulants, and cardiac glycosides e.g. digoxin. Klabunde (2008) notes that alpha or beta blockade alters the response of epinephrine. In other words, if low doses of epinephrine are administered concurrently with alpha- blockers, the unopposed beta-2-blockade will lead to hypotensive response secondary to systemic vasodilation despite the cardiac stimulation due to beta-1 activation (Klabunde, 2008). Many patients suffering cardiac arrest take several antihypertensives i.e. clonidine, an alpha blocker, as well as antiarrhythmics i.e. propranolol, a beta-blocker.

Many patients with cardiac disease take diuretics, e.g. Lasix, which can lead to hypotension and electrolyte imbalance secondary to diuresis. If co-administered with vasopressin, furosemide increases urine flow 9-fold (FDA, n.d.). This, in addition to electrolyte depletion brought on by diuresis, could have detrimental consequences for the patient. The latter, especially hypo/hyperkalemia and hypomagnesemia, can lead to fatal arrhythmias.

Coadministration of CCBs and amiodarone can lead to additive effects including exacerbated hypotension. Coadministration of digoxin and amiodarone and epinephrine can lead to digitalis toxicity, which can lead to further serious arrhythmias (FDA, n.d.). Coadministration of Coumadin and amiodarone can lead to increased serum levels leading to increased INR levels, which puts the patient at increased risk for bleeding (Giardina & Passman, 2012).

Conclusion

Heart disease remains the leading cause of death internationally. Cardiac arrest can lead to cardiac death as well as cerebral death, systemic ischemia, organ hypoperfusion, and shock. Physiological changes occur immediately after onset of cardiac arrest, and immediate intervention is crucial to prevent long-term complications including death. An overwhelming amount of research and evidence exists; however, in order to make a sound decision regarding drug administration in the case of a cardiac arrest, etiology, comorbidities, in-hospital versus out-of-hospital cardiac arrest, and type of rhythm pre cardiac arrest must be considered. None of the drugs that can be administered during cardiac arrest has proven to increase long-term survival; however, given the severity of a cardiac arrest, immediate response is needed and for this reason, it is suggested to continue utilizing current ACLS algorithms including administration of ACLS drugs. All ACLS drugs have side effects and most have minor to severe drug-drug interactions, this is especially true for amiodarone. That being said, no long term studies with respect to adverse effects of IV amiodarone exist and once again, risks versus reward must be considered. Ideally, knowing pre-cardiac arrest rhythm, comorbidities, current medication, and electrolyte levels of the patient would help in determining which ACLS drugs should be given versus held. This; however, is an unrealistic expectation and quite impossible in the out-of-hospital setting. After reviewing available literature, the author of this essay suggests administering vasopressin as the first dose if rhythms indicate administering vasopressin or epinephrine, as vasopressin certainly will not affect a patient's chance of survival. Given the high failure rate of lidocaine, amiodarone, despite potential side effects, should remain first-line treatment of incessant VF and VT. Above all, health care professionals should be trained and understand the importance of high-quality CPR and early defibrillation as this gives the patient the best chance of survival. In the case of JG, vasopressors followed by amiodarone for shock-resistant VF/VT should be administered. Consideration should be given to the length of code with respect to prolonged resuscitation efforts and associated long-term complications to include irreversible heart dysfunction as well as brain injury.

References

AHA (2012). *Cardiac arrest statistics*. Retrieved from

    http://www.heart.org/HEARTORG/General/Cardiac-Arrest-

    Statistics_UCM_448311_Article.jsp

AHA (2010). 2010 International consensus on cardiopulmonary resuscitation and emergency

    cardiovascular care science with treatment recommendations. *Circulation (122)*.S345-

    S421. doi: 10.1161/CIRCULATIONAHA.110.971051

Aung, K., Htay, T. (2005). Vasopressin for cardiac arrest: A systemic review and meta-analysis.

    *Archives of Internal Medicine (165)*1, 17-24. doi: 10.1001/archinte.165.1.17

Boyd, T., & Brady, W. (2012). The "Code Drugs in Cardiac Arrest"—the use of cardioactive

    medications in cardiac arrest resuscitation. *The American Journal of Emergency*

    *Medicine. (30)*5, 811-818. doi: 10.1016/j.ajem.2011.04.009

FDA. (n.d.) *Amiodarone hydrochloride injection* [label]. Retrieved

    from http://www.accessdata.fda.gov/drugsatfda_docs/label/2013/075955s015lbl.pdf

FDA. (n.d.) *Epinephrine injection* [label]. Retrieved from

    http://www.accessdata.fda.gov/drugsatfda_docs/label/2012/204200s000lbl.pdf

FDA. (n.d.) *Lidocaine* [label]. Retrieved from

    http://www.accessdata.fda.gov/drugsatfda_docs/label/2014/018388s084lbl.pdf

FDA. (n.d.) *Vasopressin* [label]. Retrieved from

    http://www.accessdata.fda.gov/drugsatfda_docs/label/2014/204485Orig1s000lbl.pdf

Giardina, E. G., & Passman, R., (2014). *Clinical uses of amiodarone*. Retrieved from

    http://www.uptodate.com/contents/clinical-uses-of-amiodarone

Klabunde, R. (2009). *Cardiovascular Physiology Concepts*. Philadelphia, PA: Lippincott

    Williams & Wilkins

Mauermann, W.J., Pulido, J.N., Barbara, D.W., Abel, M.D., Li, Z., Meade, L.A., Schaff, H.V., &
White, R.D. (2012). Amiodarone versus lidocaine and placebo for the prevention of
ventricular fibrillation after aortic crossclamping: A randomized, double-blind, placebo-
controlled trial. *The Journal of Thoracic and Vascular Surgery (144)*5, 1229-34 . doi:
10.1016/j.jtcvs.2012.06.039

Oberweis, B. (2011). Is vasopressin indicated in the management of cardiac arrest? *Clinical
Correlations.* Available from http://www.clinicalcorrelations.org/?p=3828

Somberg, J.C., Bailin, S.J., Haffajee, C.I., Paladino, W.P., Kerin, N.Z., Bridges, D.,… & Molnar,
J. (2002). Intravenous lidocaine versus intravenous amiodarone (in a new aqueous
formulation) for incessant ventricular tachycardia. *The American Journal of Cardiology
(90)*8, 853-9. doi: 10.1016/S0002-9149(02)02707-8

Stroumpoulis, K., Xanthos, T., Rokas, G., Kitsou, V. (2008). Vasopressin and epinephrine in the
treatment of cardiac arrest: An experimental study. *Critical Care (12)*2, R40. doi:
10.1186/cc6838

Wenzel, V., Krismer, A.C., Arntz, H.R., Sitter, H., Staldbauer, K. H., & Lindner, K. (2004). A
comparison of vasopressin and epinephrine for out-of-hospital cardiopulmonary
resuscitation. *The New England Journal of Medicine (350)*2, 105-113. doi:
10.1056/NEJMoa025431

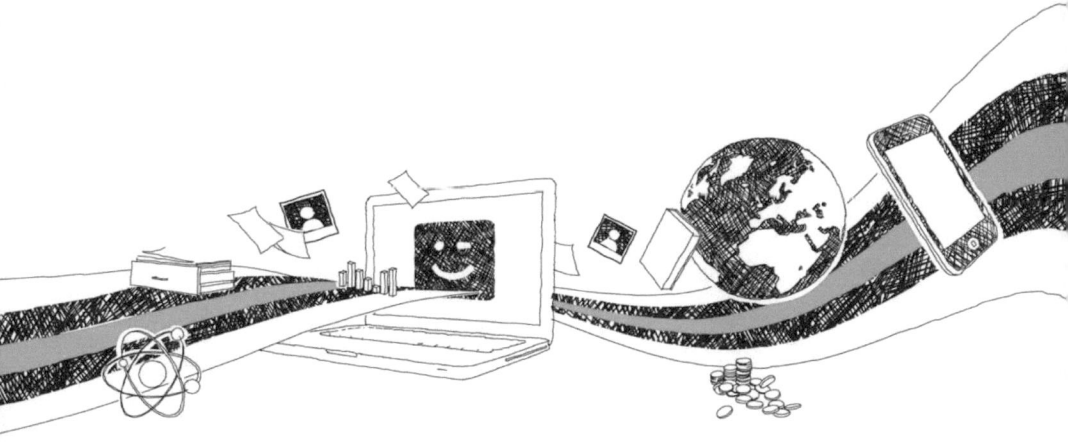
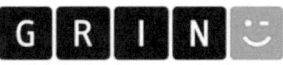